INTRODUCTION

Hey!

Welcome to **Power Your Mind: Tools to Build Resilience**, a guide for students—just like you—trying to get through their day without losing their cool.

A lot of times, the little things add up.

Maybe you are running late to meet your friends, or a teacher snapped at you, or you bombed an exam; maybe things aren't going well at home, or you are on the outs with your partner, or someone posted something nasty about you online.

Maybe you are having a **REALLY** bad day and it is all of the above, all at the same time. When these things happen, they leave us feeling a little irritated, upset, or saddened.

And, that can add up, too, leading to feelings of anxiety, anger, or depression. We lose our temper or start getting blue, and it all can spin out of control fast, making the situation worse and leaving us hurt and confused.

Power Your Mind is based on a program that has helped thousands of individuals around the world cope with events that trigger symptoms and upset. It's a tried and true method that has helped people lead more peaceful and productive lives, and it can help you handle situations that are confusing or upsetting.

This is a self-guided, self-paced guide to work through on your own, or to do as part of a group. Each section presents tools you can use to deal with everyday stress and upsets. In the pages ahead you will learn:

- That your temper has two faces and what you can do about each.
- How to recognize situations outside of yourself and better manage your inner thoughts and emotions.
- Lots of tools to deal with situations as they arise.
- The Four-Step Method for handling an event.
- And, much more!

You will find plenty of opportunities to put these lessons to the test! We'll show examples of these ideas in action and then offer tips for you to put to use in your daily life. Based on some of the programs that we have run before, we suggest you complete one session per week so you have time to think about new terms and practice.

You may be tempted to read the whole book cover-to-cover in one sitting, maybe even in one day, but we encourage you to then go back and do the activities. In order to really get the most out of this program, you should give yourself the chance to truly learn these tools. Take your time. Let things sink in. Then apply them to your life.

Before we dive into our first lesson, think about what you want to accomplish by the time you finish this guide. Look at how this program has helped others in their comments on the next page. See if any of these are familiar to you. Are you dealing with a similar situation at home?

Endorsements

"We have peace in our family today, and my family trusts me again." – Antonio

"I can see the viewpoint of others and am less sensitive to criticism." – Sara

"I don't know what I would do without this program. I had no tools to deal with my anxiety, and was barely functioning until I started learning the method." – Louise

"I think before I speak. I get less irritated and angry. I am more self-forgiving." – Lily

"This has changed my life. It has helped me grow as a person. I learned how to cope with my nervous symptoms and it taught me how to change my thoughts and see my anxiety differently." – Brendan

"It has helped me feel less anxious and more in control of my feelings and thoughts. I behave better. My family and friends notice and they find many of the tools very useful for themselves." – Tamika

Looking over this list, what resonates with you? Circle some words above that stand out, that are important to you for the future.

Setting a personal goal

Write a statement that reads like the success stories above for yourself. What do you want to improve on? What would you like to say about yourself one day?

_____

_____

_____

_____

_____

_____

_____

_____

In the weeks ahead, refer back to this page. Look at your goals and consider how you are making progress.

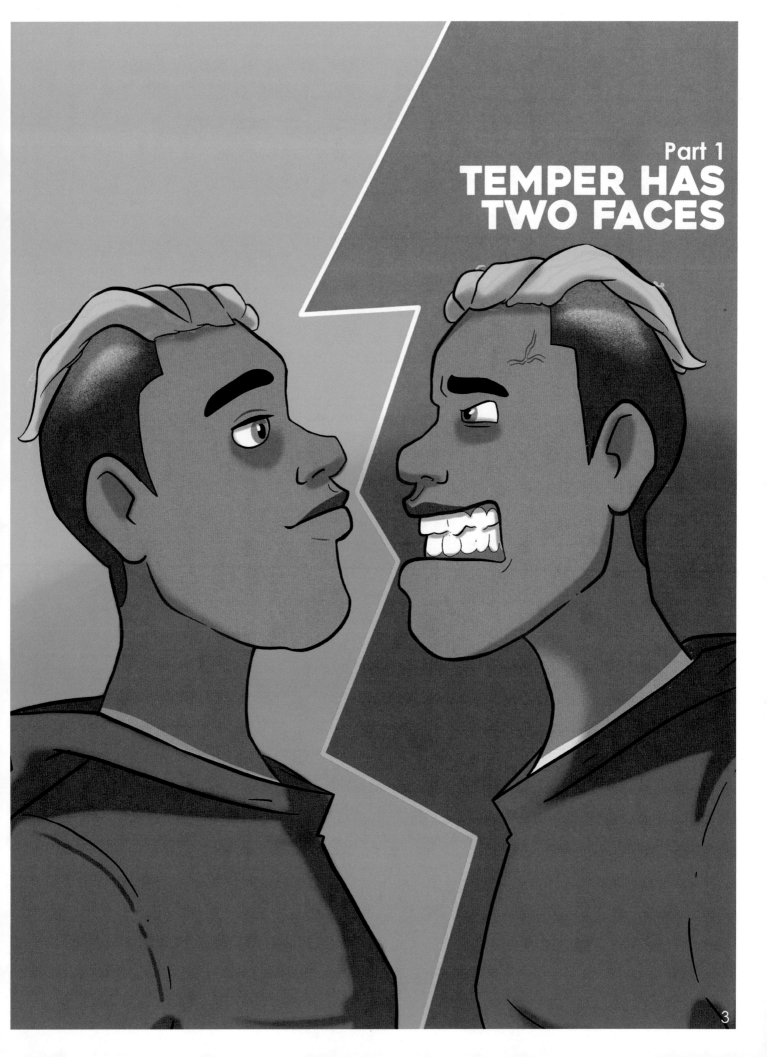

Part 1
TEMPER HAS
TWO FACES

3

TEMPER HAS TWO FACES

IN THIS SECTION YOU WILL DISCOVER

1. Temper has two faces: Angry & Fearful
2. "Judgment" is an important element of each
3. There are tools you can use to control our temper

There are two kinds of tempers.

Angry Temper is when we feel **wronged by someone else**. For example, a friend stands us up, we get cheated out of a deal, someone else gets us in trouble, or we get snubbed outright. This situation can leave us feeling irritated, resentful, disgusted, or impatient.

Fearful Temper is when we feel **we are in the wrong**. For example, we get confused about what time we are supposed to meet someone and show up late, we act silly at a party and hurt someone's feelings, or we answer a question wrong and get called out by the teacher. As a result, this can leave us feeling bad about ourselves. We start worrying, experience feelings of shame and fear, or feel hopeless.

Judgment is one thing that both types of temper have in common.

With **Angry Temper**, we are *judging* that another person has wronged us. We may not have all the facts or know the details, but we *feel* that we are right, they are wrong and act accordingly. We get **angry** when we think **other people are wrong** or **they have wronged us**.

With **Fearful Temper**, we worry that others have *judged* us as being wrong, or we *judge* ourselves as being wrong. This can make us feel self-conscious, inadequate, or ashamed.

If we could all learn to "drop the judgement," we would avoid a lot of pain and aggravation! But, it's not quite that simple.

THERE ARE TWO KINDS OF TEMPER

We can't always tell the difference when we are in it—fists balled, teeth gritted, shoulders tensed—but we can learn to spot each of them.

And, if we can identify temper, we can do something about it.

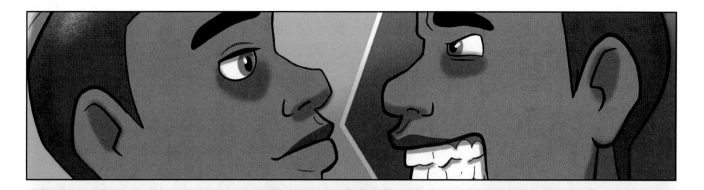

FEARFUL TEMPER

The judgment that **I am wrong**

Feelings related to Fearful Temper:
- WORRY
- FEELING OF INADEQUACY
- HOPELESSNESS
- FEAR OF DAMAGE TO YOURSELF OR YOUR REPUTATION
- SENSE OF SHAME

Can you think of more?

ANGRY TEMPER

The judgment that the **other person is wrong** or has wronged me

Feelings related to Angry Temper:
- IRRITATION
- RESENTMENT
- IMPATIENCE
- HATRED
- DISGUST
- REBELLION

Can you think of more?

HERE IS THE THING...

We can't control how other people act.

We can't really control other people at all.

We can't control events or circumstances or situations.

We can only control ourselves—and how we respond to these things.

If we think others are wrong, we get angry or rebellious.

If we think that we are wrong or others think we are wrong, we worry, feel inadequate, and feel worthless.

But we can change our reactions by controlling our thoughts, emotions, and impulses. This program will teach you how. It begins by knowing the difference between angry and fearful temper. Let's see if we can spot the temper in the story on the next page.

MEET MAX

He is waiting near the theater for his friend. See if you can figure out the kind of temper on display.

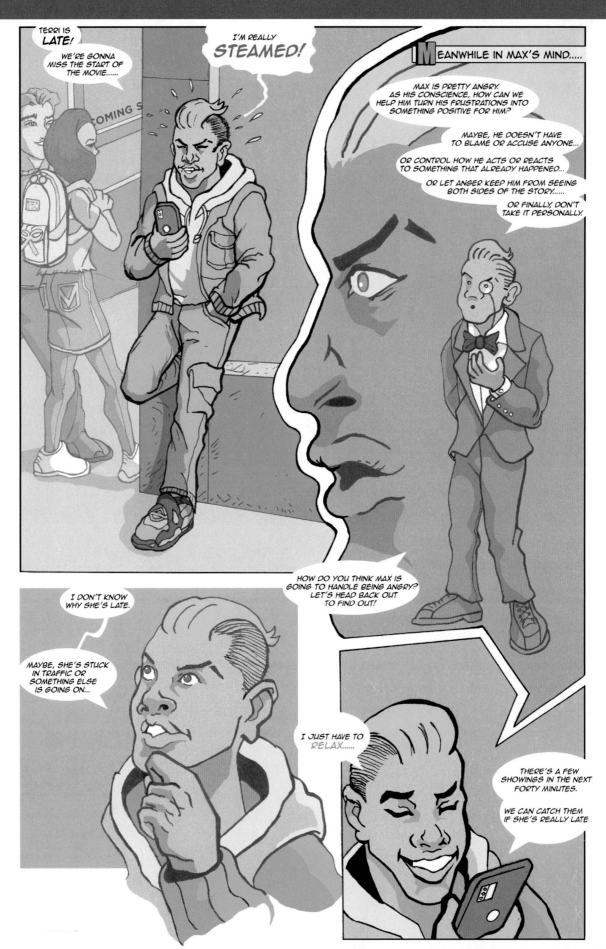

REFLECT

Let's start by unpacking Max's experience.

1. Can you tell which kind of temper (angry or fearful) Max is experiencing?
2. What does Max seem to be feeling?
3. Describe the situation.

If you said that Max was exhibiting an Angry Temper, getting irritated and impatient with Terri—you are correct.

We'll talk more about how Max handled the situation in a bit, but first, let's talk about you. In this next activity, write about a time that you thought another person was wrong and you were right. Be brief, but cover what you were feeling. How did you act? What was the experience like for you?

ACTIVITY #1

Angry Temper: Describe a time when you thought another person was wrong and you were right—this is Angry Temper:

_____

_____

_____

_____

_____

_____

_____

_____

_____

_____

_____

_____

_____

_____

In Max's situation, we saw that he was able to get his angry temper under control.

- Can you identify three ways that Max was able to keep his anger in check?
- What did Max do to calm himself down?
- How was he able to take control of the situation?

By recognizing that he didn't know both sides of the story, Max was able to manage his emotions a bit better. In addition, by identifying the situation as something relatively trivial, he was able to relax. He opted not to take it personally—he assumed Terri was not late on purpose to irritate him. He managed to calm down, and also found alternative solutions if Terri arrived too late to make the first show.

In the box below, you will see the tools that Max used, as well as other tools for managing angry temper. As you read through them, see which apply to Max's situation.

Some Tools for Angry Temper

- We can learn to express our feelings without temper.
- We excuse rather than accuse ourselves and others.
- Humor is our best friend, temper is our worst enemy.
- We choose peace over power.
- It takes two to fight, one to lay down the sword.
- If we can't change a situation, we can change our attitude toward it.
- Calm begets calm, temper begets temper.
- We drop the judgment.
- Feelings should be expressed and temper suppressed.
- Every act of self-control leads to a sense of self-respect.
- People do things *that* annoy us, usually not *to* annoy us.
- We can control our mouth and speech.
- We can remove ourselves from a tense situation.
- Temper keeps us from seeing the other side of the story.

Okay, let's look at the situation you wrote out earlier. Look at the event you listed and try to create a positive outcome (even if it didn't end that way) by using some of the tools listed above.

Choose **three** tools from this list and apply it to your own situation.

1. How could the outcome be different using these tools?
2. How can you use these tools the next time you are in a similar situation for a positive outcome?
3. What tools on the list are you committed to trying next time? Circle them. You could also take a picture of the tools on your phone for quick access.

In our next activity, let's do the same for the other kind of temper.

Remember, fearful temper occurs when you judge yourself to be wrong, or worry others are judging you to be wrong. This can lead to feelings of worry, fear, and shame. Think of a situation where this was true for you and write it below.

ACTIVITY #2

Fearful Temper: Describe a time when you thought you might be wrong, and others might be right—this is Fearful Temper:

_____

_____

_____

_____

_____

_____

_____

_____

_____

Now, let's look at ways you could have changed this situation or taken control of it for yourself. Here is a list of tools for fearful temper. As you read through the list, imagine how you could use these tools in your situation.

Some Tools for Fearful Temper

- Humor is our friend, temper is our enemy.
- We learn not to take ourselves too seriously.
- We excuse rather than accuse ourselves and others.
- This is distressing, but not dangerous.
- Calm begets calm, temper begets temper.
- Helplessness is not hopelessness.
- Temper maintains and intensifies symptoms.
- Have the courage to make mistakes.
- Fear is a belief and beliefs can be changed.
- We can accept or reject thoughts that come to us.
- Decide, plan and act.
- When feeling overwhelmed, do things in "part acts"—one step at a time.

Can you identify some of the tools you could have used? Look at the event you wrote out and try to create a positive outcome using the tools listed above.

Choose **three** tools from this list and apply it to your own situation.

1. How could the outcome be different using these tools?
2. How can you use these tools the next time you are in a similar situation for a positive outcome?
3. What tools on the list are you committed to trying next time?

In our next chapter, we'll visit Terri and see what she can teach us about our internal and external environment, but first, let's review what you learned in this section.

REVIEW

Now that you have finished this section, you should be able to:

1. Tell the difference between the two types of temper. Angry Temper is when we feel wronged by someone else. Fearful Temper is when we feel we are in the wrong.

2. Recognize Angry and Fearful Temper in your own experiences.

3. Identify some tools for each type of temper and have a plan to use them.

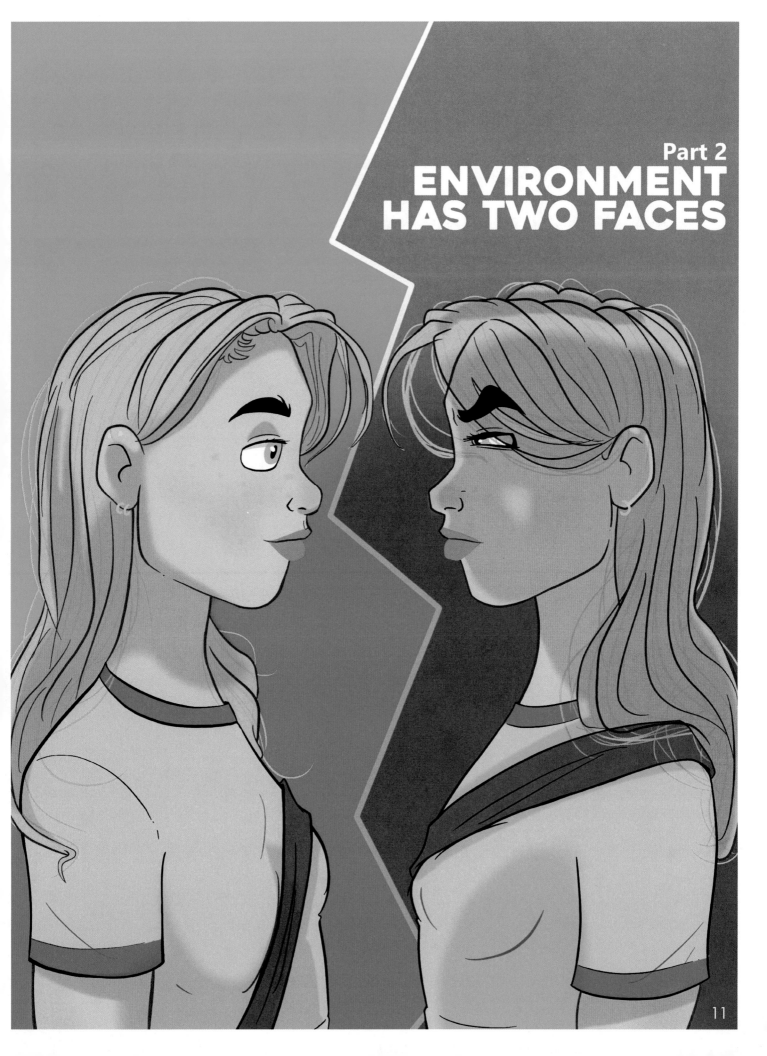

Part 2

ENVIRONMENT HAS TWO FACES

IN THIS SECTION YOU WILL DISCOVER

1. Environment has two faces: Internal & External
2. The difference between the two
3. What you can do to deal with each

We can't control what our friends or family do. We can't control our partner or significant other. We can't control the guy on the bus or the woman in the next car.

No matter how much we want them to behave a certain way—it is quite literally, out of our hands, or beyond our fingertips.

Same with events.

We may want something to happen—to make the team, get a part in the school play, or land that afterschool job—but once we've done our part (try out, audition, or apply) those things are out of our control and in the hands of other people.

That is also true for accidents, world events, things we watch online, or catch on TV. We can't control these outcomes.

Finally, you can't control the past any more than you can control people or events. Your history is beyond your fingertips.

Whatever has happened. Experiences in your childhood. Memories. History. These things are also outside of your control. It's over, even if you think about them once in a while.

Okay, before you throw your hands up and surrender— "*Forget about it, everything is out of my control*"—let's talk about what you *can* do.

HOLD YOUR HAND OUT IN FRONT OF YOU.

GO AHEAD.

Hold it at chest level, shoulder height, looking at your fingertips.

Right there, the tips of your fingers—that is also the edge of your control—the end of it.

It is easy to forget, but we can't control anything outside our skin.

People. Events. Our past.

We can't control these things. These are our outer **(external) environment**.

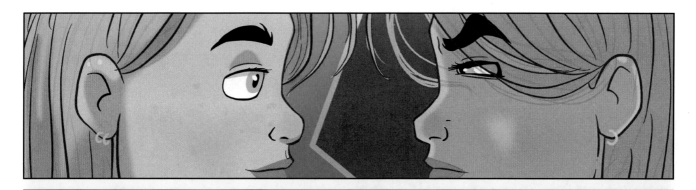

Inner (Internal) Environment

You **CAN'T** control any of these:

- FEELINGS
- SENSATIONS

You **CAN** control these:

- THOUGHTS
- IMPULSES

Outer (External) Environment

Everything outside your skin
You **CAN'T** control any of these:

- PEOPLE
- EVENTS
- THE PAST

TRY THIS...

Flip your hands over so that the palms face up, and the back of the hand points toward the ground.

Curl those fingers inward in a ball, so that the fingertips point back at yourself. Almost everything inside your skin, your **inner (internal) environment** is within your control.

You can control your thoughts. You can control your impulses. You can control your actions and reactions. You can control your own muscles and movements.

That is the most important thing to take away from this lesson.

Your initial feelings and sensations—the startle or immediate reaction to an event—are natural, inborn, and not controllable. BUT, the next response—how you react to these emotions, feelings, sensations—is completely under your control.

You can only control what is in your control.

MEET TERRI

Terri is on her way to meet Max. She is running late. And Max is probably going to be upset with her. Check out what is going through her head as she sits in traffic.

See if you can tell the difference between her inner environment—*what she can control*—and her outer environment—*what is outside her control.*

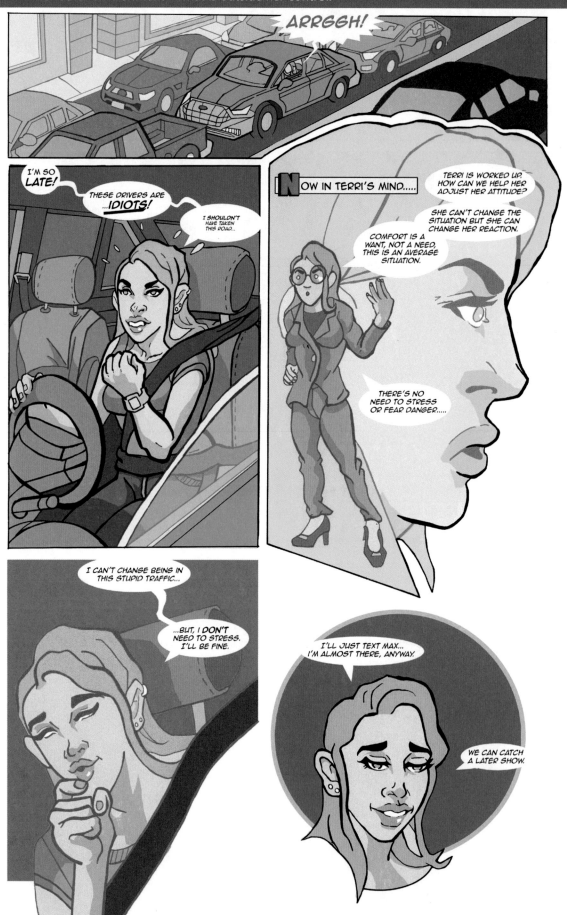

REFLECT

Let's start by unpacking Terri's experience.

1. Can you tell what is part of her internal environment?
2. Can you tell what is external?
3. What is in Terri's control?
4. How can she manage her response?
5. Describe the situation.

Terri can't control the time, the traffic, other drivers on the road, or whether or not Max is mad at her.

We've been there, right?

We are going to meet a friend, heading to practice, or running late for class, and everything feels overwhelming. We make the situation worse by giving in to our emotions and panicking.

What Terri **can** control is how she responds to these other people and events. She feels anxious and frustrated, but she smooths things out by talking herself down and taking action. She acknowledges what is not in her control, recognizes what is, and sends Max a text.

ACTIVITY #1

Look around and name three things you see in the **external** environment that you can't control:

_____

Name three feelings or sensations you have right now in your **internal** environment that you can't control: (are you nervous, worried, angry, achy, sad?)

_____

Name three thoughts or impulses you have right now that you **can** control:
(might you laugh, or roll your eyes?)

_____

ACTIVITY #2

Describe a stressful event. The last time you were into it with your parents or your friends. Describe the situation. Pay special attention to what was going on **outside your control**, what was happening internally (feelings, sensations, thoughts), and how you dealt with each:

_____

_____

_____

_____

_____

Now, let's combine the concepts of **temper and environment.** Look at Max's situationl. He was angry. He could also have been insecure, thinking that Terri didn't care about him enough to be on time. By recognizing his inner feelings of **angry** or **fearful temper** and **using tools**, then Max changed his thoughts, stayed calm, and gained control.

When we feel anxious about an everyday situation that we can't get out of—like Terri stuck in traffic—we can **spot angry temper** (frustration at others). Then using the **tools**, _"If we can't change a situation, we can change our attitude towards it"_ and _"we can take a secure thought"_ that it won't last forever, we can take control of the situation.

The same situation could turn to **fearful temper** by accusing ourselves with thoughts like, _"I should have left the house earlier"_ or _"I shouldn't have come this way."_ Again, this is a time to remember tools like, _"I spot that it is average to get caught in traffic,"_ _"this is distressing but not dangerous,"_ or _"drop the judgment."_

By using tools, we can calm ourselves down and realize that bad traffic or being late to the movies are trivial, little things—they are not emergencies. There may also be reasons we are not aware of yet: our friend may have had a flat tire, or lost track of time, or traffic may have been slow. Regardless of the reason, we can change our reactions and our plans and still enjoy time together.

ACTIVITY #3

Look at the event you wrote out and try to create a positive outcome (even if it didn't end that way) by using some of the tools listed earlier.

1. Choose **three** tools from Part 1 and apply them to your own situation.
2. How could the outcome be different using these tools?
3. How can you use these tools the next time you are in a similar situation for a positive outcome?
4. What tools on the lists are you committed to trying next time?

In our next chapter, we'll learn how to deal with things inside and outside ourselves. We will understand how to use our **will** to gain perspective, find patience, and persevere. We'll learn about self-endorsement, trivialities, and even more tools to get control of yourself, deal with situations, and respond with action.

REVIEW

In this section, we learned some valuable lessons on how to deal with everyday experiences and average events without losing your cool. Finishing this section, you should be able to tell the following:

1. The two faces of environment: internal and external.

2. How to tell the difference between them and recognize what you can control (hint: it ends at your fingertips).

3. Tools you can use to control what is in your control and let go of the rest.

NOTES & THOUGHTS

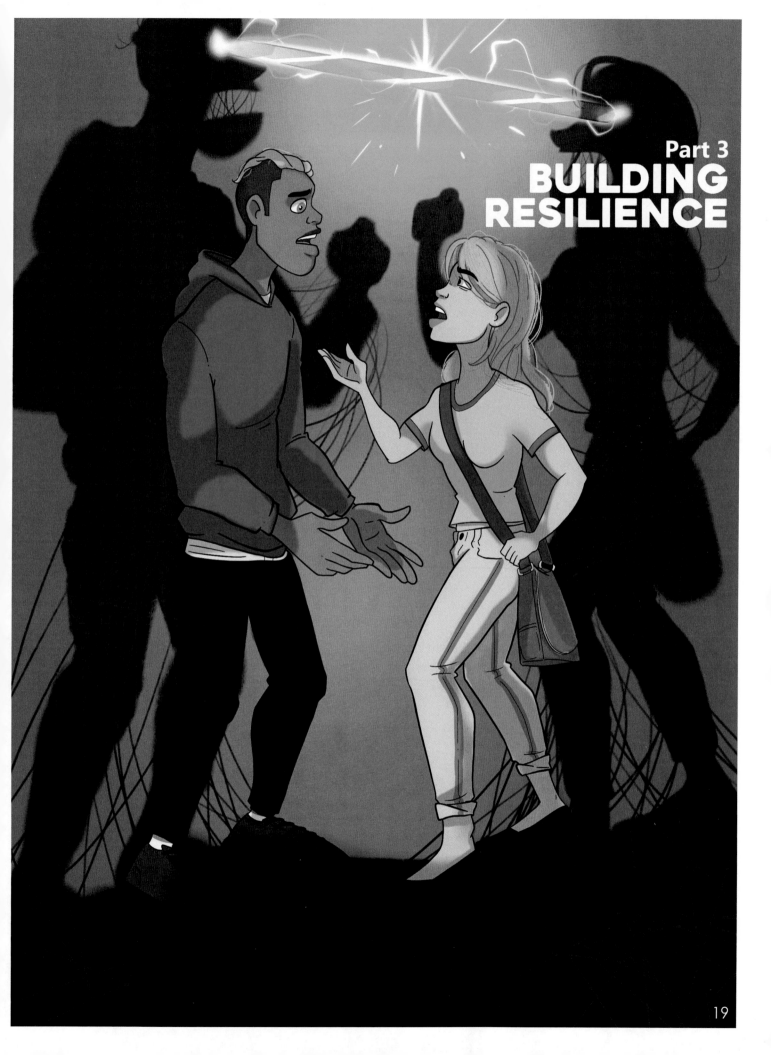

Part 3
BUILDING RESILIENCE

BUILDING RESILIENCE

IN THIS SECTION YOU WILL DISCOVER

1. Recognizing and dealing with Trivialities

2. The 3 Ps for developing the power of our Will

3. The meaning of Self-Endorsement and putting it into practice

---

Welcome back!

Things are about to get intense. We are going to define **trivialities**, those everyday events that get us upset. We are going to learn the importance of **will-power**— what it is, how to use it, and how to make it stronger. We are going to learn the power of **self-endorsement**.

Let's begin.

Will

Remember what we discussed in the last chapter—you can only control your thoughts and impulses. You cannot control other people. You cannot control a situation. In this chapter, we are going to talk about the most important thing there is to control: yourself. Being able to control your actions, emotions and impulses—that's your will.

By controlling our reactions, we can often influence the outer environment and others. For example, when we use tools to drop our temper, our calm reaction can help calm the reactions of those around us.

The tools in this program will help you act and think differently than before. If you practice them again and again, then everyday annoyances—trivialities—will not bother you as much.

And when you do that, you deserve a pat on the back!

RESILIENCE IS THE ABILITY TO BOUNCE BACK, TO STAY CALM, TO RECOVER QUICKLY.

Most things that upset us are little things. If we learn to manage our responses to life's trivial events, we'll cope better and stay calm. And, we'll be better able to handle big challenges when they arise.

Self-control—having the will to choose a positive response in a situation—is key to building resilience.

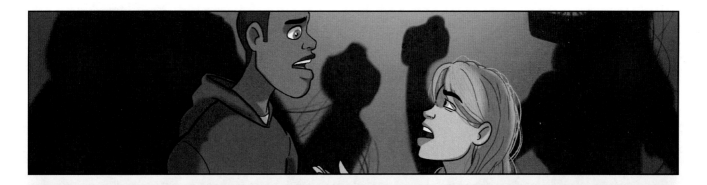

TRIVIALITIES

Most things that upset us are the routine events in everyday life.

YOUR WILL

You have the power to choose:

- HOW YOU ARE GOING TO ACT
- WHAT YOU ARE GOING TO THINK

SELF-ENDORSEMENT

You deserve a mental pat on the back for any effort:

- TO SPOT YOUR TEMPER
- TO CONTROL YOUR THOUGHTS AND IMPULSES

The 3Ps for Developing our Will

Think of will-power like a muscle. Strengthening your will builds resilience.

In the same way that you make yourself stronger by lifting weights, faster by running, or more flexible by doing yoga—we can have more self-control by exercising our *will*.

We exercise our will through 3Ps.
Perseverance. Patience. Perspective.

- *The will to persevere*— that means grit. Finding a way to keep going when we feel beat down and stick with something until it's finished.

- *The will to patience*— we know that one, it just means finding a "pause" button. Stopping our emotional response, so we can catch our breath and get some clarity.

- *The will to get perspective*— this is the moment when you choose how to think or respond.

Next, we'll meet Cheryl, who needs to maintain perspective in order to remain calm in an average, everyday situation.

Cheryl is shopping at the mall when she sees a friend. She calls out, but her friend doesn't respond.

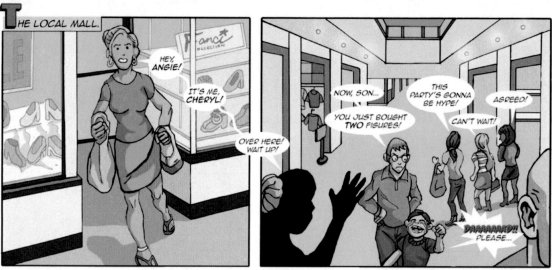

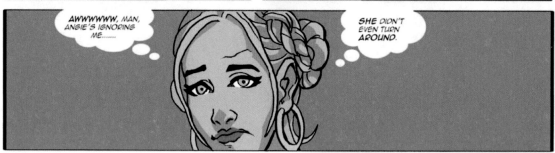

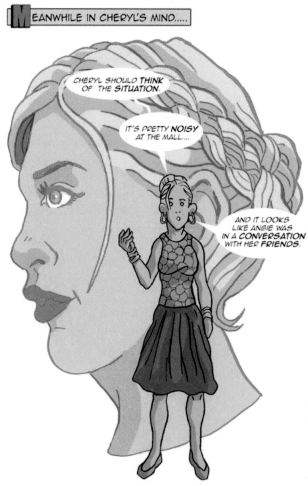

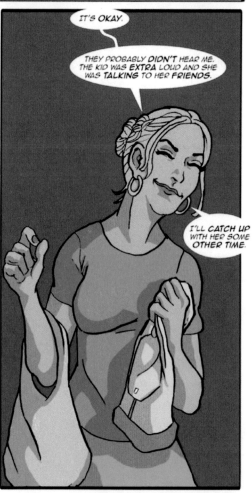

REFLECT

Might Cheryl have felt angry, blaming others for making so much noise that her friend didn't hear her? Or might she have felt upset—fearful temper—that her friend might have ignored her on purpose, dissing her? Either way, she might be feeling bad—wanting to yell or tear up.

Instead, she used her tools to recognize this wasn't a big deal. She recognized she couldn't control the situation—it was noisy—and she excused her friend for not hearing her. So instead of yelling louder and making a scene, or hanging her head as if she'd been shunned, she shrugged it off and went on her way.

Trivialities are things that happen in everyday life. They are not right or wrong, they just happen. We give them value with our thoughts, emotions, and actions. We can choose how we respond to them. We can let them get us worked up and frustrated or we can let them go.

Some Tools for Trivialities

- Expectations can lead to disappointments.
- Sometimes people do things *that* annoy us, not *to* annoy us.
- Treat life as a business, not as a game.
- Do the thing you fear and hate to do, as long as there is no danger.
- Try, fail; try, fail; try, succeed.
- You can't control the outer environment.
- The outer environment can be rude, crude and indifferent.
- Have the courage to make a mistake in the trivialities of everyday life.
- We can't change an event, we can only change our attitude toward it.
- There is no right or wrong in the trivialities of everyday life.

Think of Terri stuck in traffic. Thinking to herself: "I shouldn't have taken this route." She is blaming herself (fearful temper) for taking the "wrong way" and blaming others (angry temper) for making the traffic so heavy. These things are trivial. Her judgments give them value—negative value, in this case.

ACTIVITY #1

Write out your day. Start from the time that you woke up until this present moment. Think of all the small events that happened between then and now. Did you brush your teeth? Did you eat breakfast? Did you get dressed? All of these actions were **trivial**. Write them out, like an after-the-fact "to-do" list—an "all-done" list!

_____   1 2 3 4 5 6 7 8 9 10

_____   1 2 3 4 5 6 7 8 9 10

_____   1 2 3 4 5 6 7 8 9 10

_____   1 2 3 4 5 6 7 8 9 10

_____   1 2 3 4 5 6 7 8 9 10

Now, go over the same list and see where you might have given an action significance—rate each event from mild (1) to intense (10). What value did you ascribe to it? Maybe picking out your clothes was difficult because you were afraid of being criticized. Or, was it easy because you wore your favorite shirt? Give it a number.

Once you've done that, look over the list of tools and see if any of them could have helped change your attitude or rating about these trivial events.

ACTIVITY #2

Will-Power: Below are tools for building our will. Circle at least three you'd like to practice this week.

Some Tools for Will

- We can decide which thoughts to think.
- We can decide which words to use.
- We can decide which actions to take.
- Do things in part acts—one step at a time.
- Every act of self-control leads to a greater sense of self-respect.
- Feelings and sensations cannot be controlled, but thoughts and impulses can.
- Replace an insecure thought with a secure thought.
- Move our muscles, change our minds.
- Try fail, try fail, try succeed!
- There are no uncontrollable impulses, only impulses that are not controlled.
- If we can't decide, any decision will steady us.
- It's not that we cannot, it's that we care not to bear the discomfort.
- Have the will to persevere.

ACTIVITY #3

Below are tools for patting yourself on your back. Circle at least three endorsements you'd like to practice this week.

Tools for Endorsing
- When you are endorsing yourself, you can't be blaming yourself.
- Endorse yourself when you spot your temper.
- We can decide which actions to take.
- Endorse yourself when you control your thoughts.
- Endorse yourself when you control your impulses.
- Congratulate yourself for the effort, not the outcome.

Moving forward, try to give yourself a congrats for something at least three times a day. It doesn't matter what others think—whether others recognize what you do or congratulate you. Don't seek endorsement from others, but always practice self-endorsement—this, too, builds resilience.

REVIEW

In this section, we unpacked the meaning of "will-power" and learned that, in the same way that exercise builds muscle, there are ways to develop our will and make it stronger. As we conclude this section, you should know how to:

1. Recognize ways to navigate the trivialities of everyday life.

2. Identify the 3Ps to Develop your Will: perseverance, patience, and perspective.

3. Congratulate yourself for small efforts, accomplishments, and successful situations.

In the next section, we will see how others have learned to deal with difficult situations with grace and humor, using a 4-step approach and the tools we are learning.

NOTES & THOUGHTS

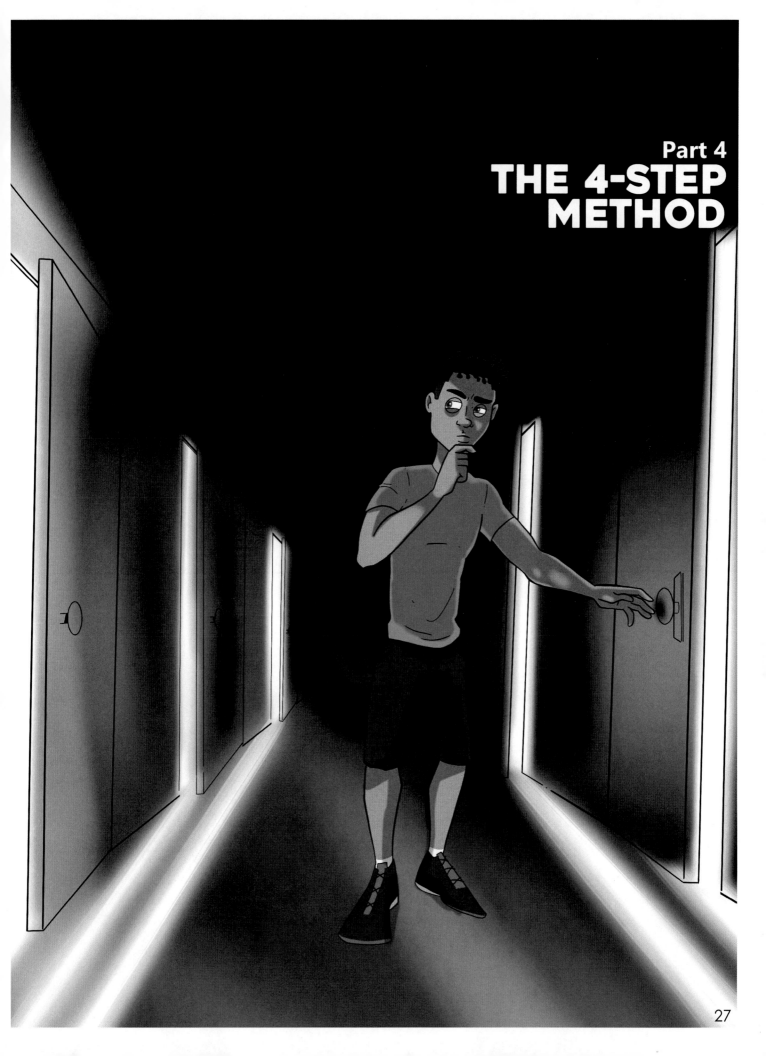

Part 4
THE 4-STEP METHOD

Part 4
THE 4-STEP METHOD

IN THIS SECTION YOU WILL DISCOVER
1. The 4-Step Method for Taking Control
2. Identifying an Event
3. Recognizing your Symptoms
4. Influencing an Outcome

Step 1 begins with an **event.**

An event is an objective experience. It is what actually occurs without our thoughts, impressions, and judgments getting in the way. Remember, in the last section, when we talked about trivialities, we recognized that experiences are only "good" or "bad" when we apply judgment to them. An event is composed of who was there, what was said, actions that were taken, and the time and place of the experience. It is everything that goes into an experience without our own perspectives layered into the event.

When we are taking the first step in the process, we describe just the facts of the event, without adding embellishments or feelings.

Step 2 in this process involves the **symptoms** we experience.

If you step off a curb to cross the street and a car blows the light and narrowly misses you, your body is going to react. Your heart might pick up its pace. You feel a sudden rush of energy flood your system. Your breath gets quick and shallow. These are symptoms, triggered by the event.

Your feelings, sensations, thoughts, and impulses (anxiety, racing heart, tight jaw, wanting to cry or yell, etc.) are all symptoms. Naming them is a way to get them in check.

Step 1: Event
Briefly describe the event: the time and place, the things that were said and done, the people involved. End with: "That's when I began to work myself up."

Step 2: Symptoms
Describe the symptoms and discomfort you experienced: your feelings, sensations, thoughts, and impulses (anxiety, racing heart, tight jaw, wanting to cry or yell.)

Step 3: Spotting
Describe if you noticed angry or fearful temper in your reaction. What tools did you use? Did you endorse?

Step 4: Outcome
Describe what would have happened before you learned these tools—the reaction and discomfort you would have experienced.

Then describe your reaction after using the tools in this workbook. This shows progress.

Endorse yourself for your effort or any improvement!

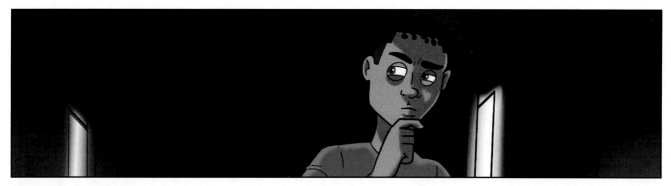

Step 3 is **spotting**.

This goes back to the first chapter: notice your temper. Is it angry or fearful?

Spotting is identifying your temper and figuring out what tools in your toolkit you need to use to get your symptoms under control.

You need to identify the parts of the external or internal environment that influence the event. What tools do you use for these? How can you look at the situation without letting things get out of control?

Step 4 is **outcome**.

This is a way of looking at the situation with different outcomes.

Imagine what the situation looks like when you put your tools in action vs. the way it looked when you didn't.

Before you learned and started practicing with the tools, your symptoms and emotions were running the show. Maybe you lost your temper when you felt insulted. Perhaps a misunderstanding led to an avoidable situation where you got in a fight with a friend and stopped talking for weeks.

Now, the same situation when you apply your tools plays out differently. You manage to recognize that your friend wasn't intentionally trying to hurt you. By keeping yourself in check and not lashing out, you keep your friendship intact and your emotions under control.

ACTIVITY #1

Remember Max from Part 1 waiting for Terri in front of the movie theater? Let's ask him to apply the **4-Step Method** to his situation.

Step 1

Describe an everyday event that got you worked up. What triggered temper and symptoms?

Max: I was waiting for a friend, and she was late. That's when I started getting worked up.

Step 2

Report the symptoms you experienced—both physical and mental.

Max: I was clenching my jaw, thinking angry thoughts, saying angry words.

Step 3

Report your fearful and angry temper, the tools you used, and self-endorsement.

Max: I was afraid she blew me off, that she didn't care to show up. I was angry she kept me waiting. I spotted that I should excuse, not accuse, that I shouldn't take it personally— maybe she couldn't help it. I endorsed for realizing I could control my reaction.

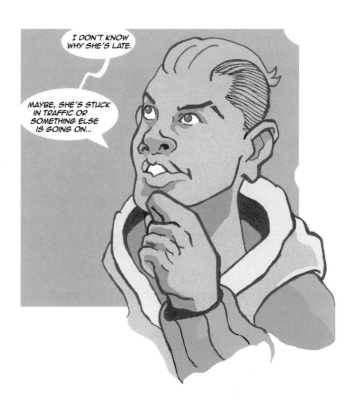

Step 4

Describe what would have happened before this training—your reaction or discomfort— and **Endorse** yourself for your effort or any improvement!

Max: Before this, I would have yelled at her when she got there, we would have fought, and it would have ruined the whole evening. Now, I could relax and figure out a plan B.

Additional Spotting of **Angry Temper**: In a support group meeting, we'd invite others to spot more tools Max could have used. Look at the tools for Angry Temper in Part 1 – what other tools do you think he could have used?

_____

_____

_____

Additional Spotting of **Fearful Temper**: Max also admits he had fearful temper—that Terri might have decided not to show up. Look at the tools for Fearful Temper in Part 1 – what other tools do you think he could have used?

_____

_____

ACTIVITY #2

Let's check out Terri's situation from Part 2 as she heads to the movie theater to see Max. How would the **4-Step Method** in help in her case?

Step 1: **Describe** Terri's situation. Where is she? What is happening? What does the event look like objectively?

_____

_____

_____

Step 2: What were Terri's **symptoms**? What was she experiencing? What was she telling herself? What was happening emotionally? Physically?

_____

_____

_____

Step 3: **Spotting:** What kind of temper was Terri experiencing? What was she thinking about the other drivers on the road? What tools listed in Parts 1- 3 did she use?

_____

_____

_____

Step 4: **Outcome:** What would have happened before Terri used the tools she'd learned? What might have happened differently in her situation with Max? Did she **endorse herself?**

_____

_____

_____

Now, let's see how Terri described her situation using the 4-Step Method. Compare your description to hers. What tempers did she spot? Did you identify different tools than she did? There are many different ways to describe any situation, and many tools that can be used. That's why we often say there is no right or wrong in trivialities—we don't have to judge that one person's answer is better than the other, because many answers and tools apply in any situation.

Step 1
I got stuck in traffic and was going to be late meeting up with Max—he hates that!

Step 2
My heart was racing, I was gripping the steering wheel. I was getting panicky.

Step 3
I was blaming myself for choosing this route, I was blaming the other drivers. I spotted this was an average situation—it could happen to anyone, and that I can't change it, but I can change how I react to it. I congratulated myself for calming down.

Step 4
Before using my tools, I would have been in tears by the time I got to Max, I would have been afraid he was mad, and it all would have been a big mess and a terrible night. Now, I am calmer, knowing it's not my fault, and hope that there's a later show we can go to.

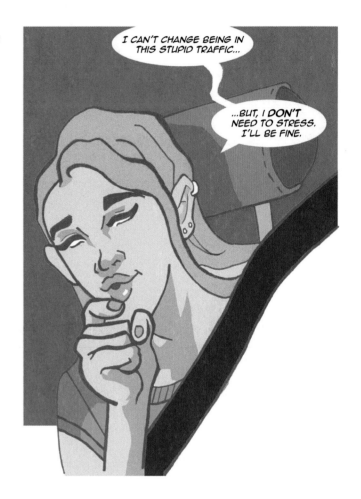

ACTIVITY #3
Now, let's look at the **4-Step Method** with an example from your own life.

Step 1: **Describe** an upsetting situation. Where are you? What is happening? What does the event look like objectively?

_____

_____

_____

_____

Step 2: **Report** the discomfort you experienced right after the event—the first signs that you were in temper. What were your feelings, impulses, sensations, and thoughts in the example you gave? *(Did your heart race? Did your jaw clench? Did you feel like yelling or crying? Were you blaming yourself or someone else?)*

_____

_____

_____

What score would you rate your discomfort on a scale of 1 to 10? (1 mild to 10 very intense)

Before Spotting: 1   2   3   4   5   6   7   8   9   10

Step 3: **Spotting** temper & tools

Look at the diagrams of Temper and Environment, and describe which you experienced:

Angry or Fearful Temper – Did you feel someone else was wrong? Were you worried you were wrong? Or that someone else might think you were wrong?

Inner or Outer Environment – Which parts of the situation were out of your control? Which were part of your inner feelings? Which parts could you control?

_____

_____

_____

_____

Look at the lists of tools, and write down which ones can help manage your reaction to this incident:

_____

_____

_____

Step 4: Describe what would have happened **before this training** and using the tools—the reaction and discomfort you would have experienced:

_____

_____

_____

Describe your reaction after using the tools in this program:

_____

_____

_____

_____

Now rate your symptoms after using the tools on a scale of 1 to 10 (1 mild to 10 very intense)

After Spotting: 1   2   3   4   5   6   7   8   9   10

Compare your "Before and After" scores and reactions.

Endorse yourself for your effort or any improvement!

REVIEW

In this section, we learned how to take control of ourselves and our actions by using the 4-Step Method. As we conclude this chapter, you should know how to:

1. Consider an event objectively— relying on just the facts of the experience to keep from overreacting.

2. Recognize our symptoms— what we are telling ourselves about the experience and what we are feeling emotionally and physically.

3. Spot the right solution that will work in a given situation.

4. Influence an outcome by considering how events might play out in response to different actions and reactions.

There are additional blank worksheets in the back of this book to write out more 4-Step Examples. Copy them, and try to write out at least three examples each week to learn the 4 Steps and the tools by heart. You can find downloadable worksheets and more tool lists at **www.poweryourmind.org.**

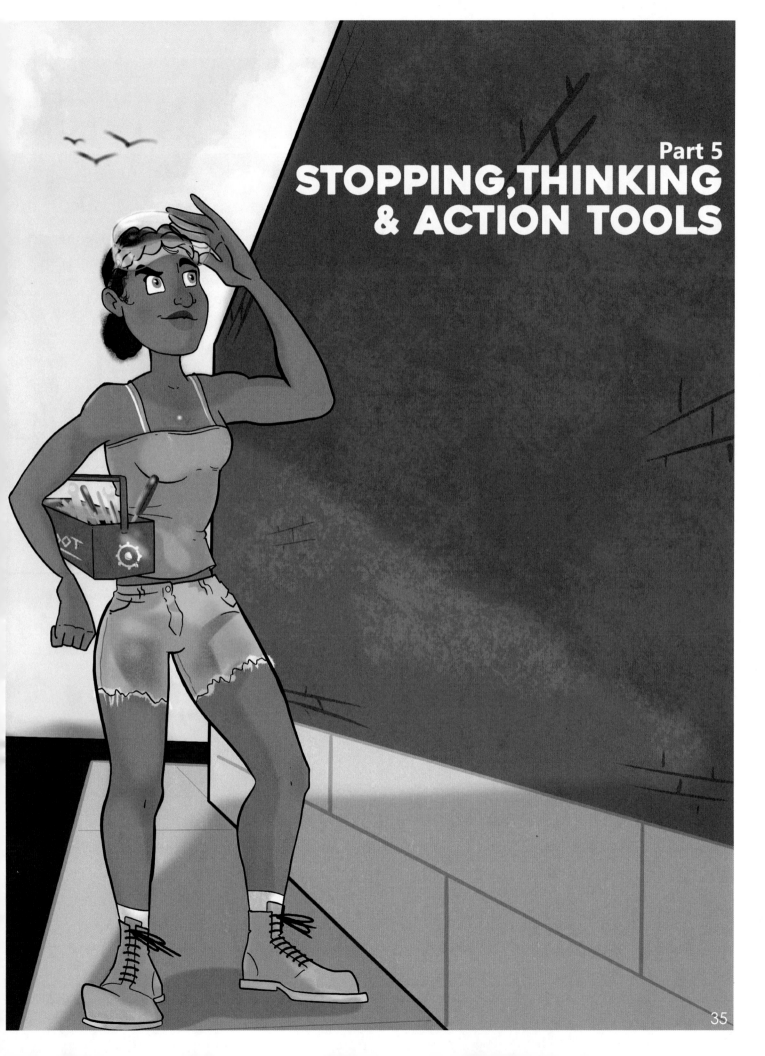

Part 5
STOPPING, THINKING & ACTION TOOLS

Part 5

STOPPING, THINKING & ACTION TOOLS

IN THIS SECTION YOU WILL DISCOVER
1. Stopping Tools
2. Thinking Tools
3. Action Tools
4. The Importance of Choice

You may have already noticed that some tools work in many different situations—using humor, for example, can help with both fearful and angry temper. Laughing at yourself is a way to cope with your internal environment and laughing at a situation is also a way to cope with the external environment.

Some tools have shown up on more than one list in previous chapters, and that's OK when you are organizing tools to deal with specific symptoms or feelings or situations.

In this section, we are going to open up the toolkit and look at three types of tools in a different way—**stopping tools, thinking tools, and action tools**—to understand what they are and how to use them. These tools can be applied to a variety of situations, but they share a common thread as they teach your brain to either stop, think, or act.

We have been talking about tools a lot throughout this workbook.

Tools for figuring out what you are feeling.

Tools for understanding your thinking.

Tools for taking action.

Tools for getting yourself under control.

Some tools teach your brain to stop doing things, some tools teach your brain to start doing different things. Learning which tools to use when is part of the process.

MEET JUAN

He has been practicing this program for more than six months.
It has helped him control his angry temper to the extent that his family and friends have noticed.

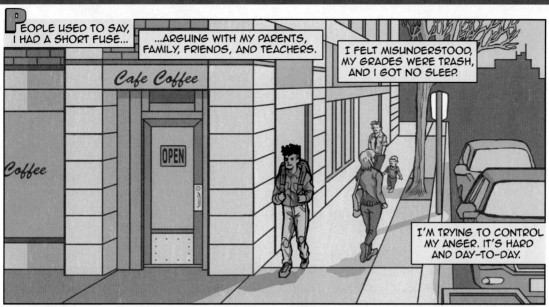

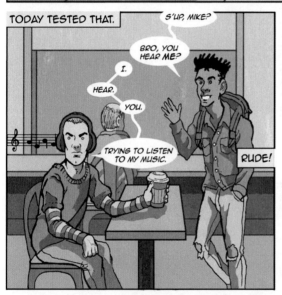

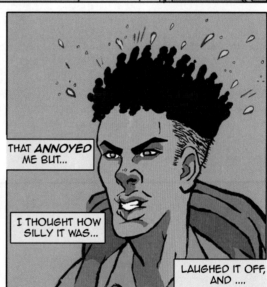

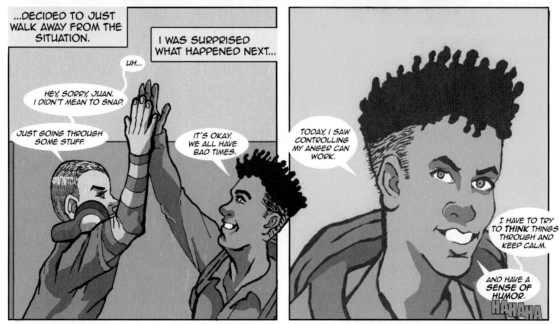

REFLECT

Juan knows he has a short fuse on his angry temper.

Being aware of this means that he can do something about it.

He uses Stopping Tools a lot—Don't judge, Don't talk, Don't accuse others.

Look at the list below—are there other stopping tools he used in this situation?

Stopping Tools

Stopping Tools help you pump the brakes before you act or react to what you are feeling or experiencing.

Stopping Tools are ways that you can hit pause between Step 2 and Step 3 in the 4-Step Method. In other words, let's say an event has occurred, we are experiencing symptoms of anger and anxiety, getting worked up, and about to react.

Stopping Tools get us out of our thoughts, out of the story we are telling ourselves, out of the moment—so we can respond more appropriately without being hijacked by our emotions.

Tools for Stopping

- Don't act.
- Don't talk.
- Don't move.
- Don't look regretfully into the past.
- Don't look fearfully into the future.
- Don't take yourself too seriously.
- Don't go for a symbolic victory.
- Don't express anti-social responses.
- Don't try to change a situation.
- Don't accuse others.
- Don't accuse yourself.
- Don't expect too much.
- Don't express temper.
- Don't avoid decisions.
- Don't expect to be perfect.
- Don't try to please everybody.
- Don't try to control others.
- Don't be selfish.
- Don't dominate.

Let's look at a couple of these more closely.

Don't act is exactly as it sounds. Often when we are getting worked up, feeling the symptoms of anger or anxiety, we want to do something about it. This stopping tool is to respond to that impulse. Rather than give over to our emotions, we choose to hit pause for a moment instead. We choose to draw a deep breath or shut our eyes and let things slide. **We stay still, we don't act.**

Don't accuse others. It is so easy to fall into the blame game. Something isn't going right. You are feeling out of sorts. In your emotions. In your head. Rather than look at the response as something you are feeling as the result of an event, you look for someone to blame. You look at the other person as responsible for your emotional state. Instead, try to look at the event objectively, realize there may be other sides to the story, get control over your response. **Don't accuse others** or yourself — judgment leads to angry or fearful temper, both in you and others.

Stopping Tools are ways that we can avoid troublesome or challenging behavior. They are actions we ***don't*** want to take.

ACTIVITY #1

Even though you just learned these tools, you probably can think of a time when you stopped yourself from doing something. Note the tool and when you used it.

Tool:

Don't _____

I recall the time when: _____

_____

_____

_____

_____

_____

Thinking Tools

Thinking Tools are for keeping things in perspective. It is so easy for thoughts to spin out of control and push us into a story we are telling ourselves about an event. We end up responding to these stories rather than the event itself.

Thinking tools help us realize that there are different ways to look at things and that there are options when choosing next steps. These give us opportunities to practice patience and perseverance.

Tools for Thinking

- Comfort is a want, not a need.
- Every act of self-control leads to a sense of self-respect.
- Expectations can lead to self-induced frustrations.
- Fear is a belief; beliefs can be changed.
- Fearful anticipation is often worse than the realization.
- Feelings and sensations cannot be controlled, but thoughts and impulses can.
- Feelings are not facts; they can lie to us.
- Feelings rise and fall.
- Frustrations are tolerable.
- Have the will to persevere.
- Helplessness is not hopelessness.
- Humor is our friend; temper is our enemy.
- Hurt feelings are just beliefs not shared.
- It is OK to feel uncomfortable in an uncomfortable situation.
- It's OK to be average.
- It takes two to fight, one to lay down the sword.
- It's not that we cannot, it's that we care not to bear the discomfort.
- Life is full of frustrations and irritations.

Let's examine two of these to understand thinking tools better.

Fearful anticipation is often worse than the realization. There is a famous quote by the writer Mark Twain that goes like this: "I've had a lot of worries in my life, most of which never happened." Worrying about something that might happen is often worse than the experience of the thing itself. This is why it is so important for us to have the facts rather than us making up a story. We need to know what is actually happening to deal with it. And, often, the outcome of something we dread—a difficult conversation, admitting we did something wrong—is often not as bad as we thought it would be.

It is OK to feel uncomfortable in an uncomfortable situation. It is, unfortunately, common for us to deny our emotions. We think that we are supposed to act a certain way. That we can't afford to be scared or angry or sad. We try to deny these negative emotions and convince ourselves that we need to just power through a situation or tough it out. Sometimes we do this at such a deep level we don't even realize we are not allowing ourselves to feel. It is okay not to feel okay.

ACTIVITY #2

Write about a situation when you really wanted to say or do something, but decided not to or that it just wasn't worth it.

_____

_____

_____

_____

_____

_____

Tools that might apply to this example:
- Every act of self-control leads to a sense of self-respect.
- Feelings and sensations cannot be controlled, but thoughts and impulses can.

Think about a time when you were in an uncomfortable situation. What were the feelings and thoughts you experienced?

_____

_____

_____

_____

_____

_____

Tools that might apply to this example:
- It is OK to feel uncomfortable in an uncomfortable situation.
- Have the will to persevere.

Action Tools

Action Tools are positive thoughts, actions, or states that you can choose for yourself. These are things you can start doing, right now, or in a challenging situation to influence the outcome. Action tools are a way to reframe your thinking and to get your brain to get your muscles moving.

Tools for Action

- Anticipate joyfully.
- Assert yourself without temper.
- Be group-minded.
- Be self-led.
- Break old habits.
- Change to secure thoughts.
- Change your attitude to the situation.
- Control your mouth.
- Decide, plan and act.
- Decide which action to take.
- Decide which thoughts to think.
- Decide which words to use.
- Do things you don't like to do.
- Do things one step at a time.
- Endorse for each effort.
- Excuse others.
- Excuse yourself.
- Express feelings.
- Have the courage to make mistakes.
- Try again.

Let's check out some action tools up close.

Assert yourself without temper. We often put our own needs aside, because we are afraid of what might happen if we actually express what we want. Maybe, we are ashamed of wanting something for ourselves. Perhaps, we are afraid someone will judge us, deny us, reject us, or hurt us for expressing what we want. Whatever our concern, denying what we want can lead us to anger without ever giving the other person a chance to do right by us! By saying what you want in a direct, straightforward, assertive way can go a long way to you getting it. When faced with someone else who is in angry temper, it is important that you do not react angrily yourself—yet you may need to assert yourself without temper.

Have the courage to make mistakes. This is a big one. We are often so scared to take action because we are afraid we are going to look stupid. We get worked up thinking that mistakes are bad and failure is wrong. It turns out though that failure is how we learn, and mistakes are part of the process of getting things right. We get so afraid about how we are going to look that we often choose not to take any action rather than move forward and make a mistake.

ACTIVITY #3

You have probably demonstrated using a few of these tools in the past. Write about a time when you had the courage to just try something new even if you had doubts about your success.

_____

_____

_____

_____

_____

_____

Tools that might apply to this example:

- Have the courage to make mistakes.
- Try again.

The Importance of Choice

Choice is the ultimate tool. It gives us the ability to act, react, or do neither. It allows us to control our thoughts. It influences outcomes. Choice is the ability to choose between the tools in our toolkit to take positive action.

If you are angry and about to yell at someone or hit them—STOP! Don't move. Don't talk. Think about what is going on. Decide whether or not to say something—calm things down rather than work them up further.

On the other hand, if you are feeling a little nervous and you want reassurance—SPEAK UP! Move your mouth and say something—ask a question or express what you want directly.

The graphic below shows how choice can influence the outcome. When something happens (an event), we react with feelings. These feelings create an impulse to act. You decide (with the power of choice) which action to take. You can choose if you act with temper or with calm, with anger or with humor. You can choose to give in to where the impulse takes us, or you can apply one of the tools on the list(s) above.

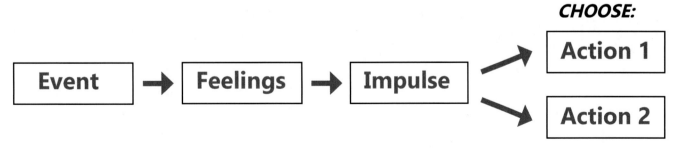

Here is the thing—**this process happens very fast.**

The speed of event to emotion to action occurs in seconds....*whoosh*...or milliseconds. Remembering you have a choice gives you power over this process.

ACTIVITY #4

Think of an event recently where you got angry or upset or overwhelmed. Write down the experience as you remember it. Make sure to be objective about it. Take the emotional story out of the event, and look at the facts.

_____

_____

_____

_____

_____

Now, write a second version of the experience where you apply what you have learned above. Apply one or two of the tools from the lists. Choose a different response. Imagine how the outcome might have changed as well.

_____

_____

_____

_____

_____

_____

REVIEW

In this section, we learned all the types of tools in our toolkit—Stopping Tools, Thinking Tools, Action Tools—to understand what they are and how to use them. As we conclude this section, you should know how to:

1. Use Thinking Tools to look at an event objectively to pull us out of the imaginative tale we are telling ourselves and look at things as they actually are.

2. Use Action Tools to move toward more positive outcomes with reframes that allow us to take action, shape our thoughts, and choose a good state of mind to move us forward. This week, practice using your three favorite tools from this chapter.

3. Use choice to create the space to influence outcomes.

Counting _choice_ as a tool, you should conclude this chapter of the workbook with ten tools in your toolkit the next time you are faced with an everyday challenging situation.

HIDDEN MEANING, HUMOR & FACING YOUR FEARS

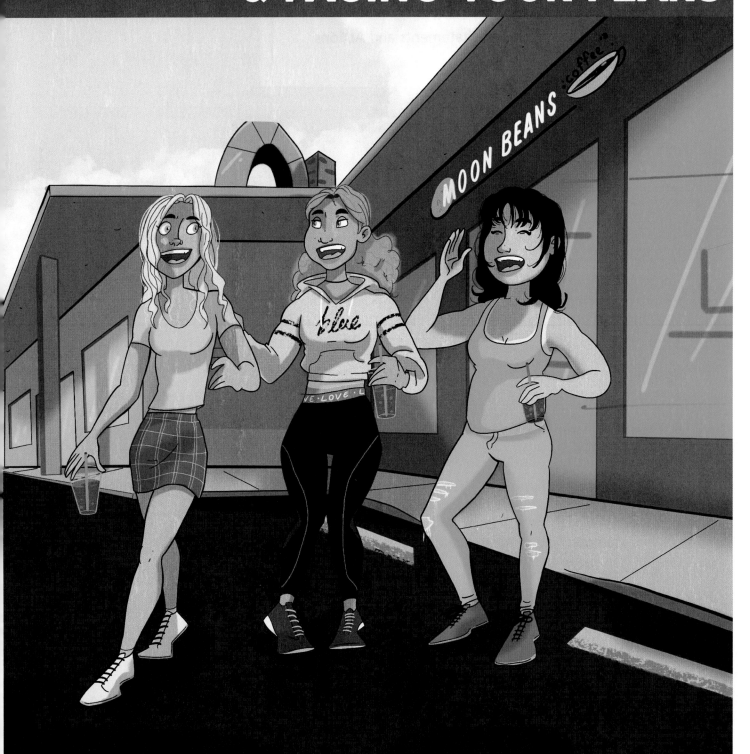

Part 6

HIDDE ... HUMOR & FACI ... ARS

KENDELA Community
210-501-2890
Daniel Hall

IN THIS SECTION YOU

1. Hidden Meanings Be
2. Humor can Defuse A
3. How to Face Your Fears

In this chapter we are going to take a deeper dive into three more crucial concepts: Hidden Meanings, Humor, and Facing Your Fears.

Through each concept, we will gain a deeper understanding of lessons presented throughout the book.

For example, *Hidden Meanings*, actually helps us deepen our understanding of **spotting**, which is an important part of the 4-Step Method. We already have a working understanding of spotting and hopefully you've been trying it out in different situations over the last couple of weeks.

Spotting often refers to finding the *meaning underneath statements and actions.*

With **surface thinking**, you can explain and express it in ordinary language.

With **intuitive thinking**, you *feel* what is underneath a statement or underneath a reaction. If you only feel it, but cannot explain why, you get angry and frustrated, you develop temper. The deeper meaning needs to become a part of your awareness.

Spotting means to look underneath statements and reactions and then be fully aware of what they mean—to recognize the intuitive thinking. Spotting allows you to learn to look into your own deeper meanings and perhaps into the deeper meanings of others around you.

We'll take a look at how this works in Gabriela's story.

art of spotting refers finding the meaning nderneath statements nd actions.

There are two kinds of thinking at work here:

1) surface thinking, refers to things that we know and can explain; and,

2) intuitive thinking, refers to things that we know but cannot explain.

The first is often easy to identify—it is the literal meaning of things. The second can be harder to see or know, but it can be done with practice and by using our tools.

MEET GABRIELA

She wants to go to the big game with her friends, and asks her mom for permission. We see her reading the hidden meaning behind mom's pauses and non-verbal body language.

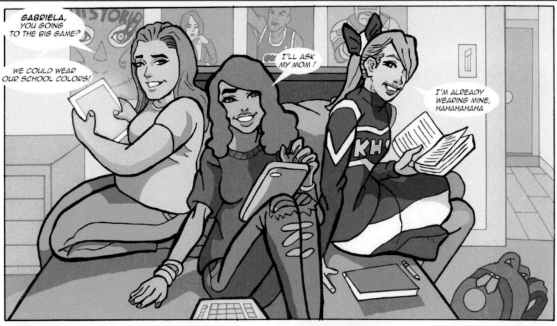

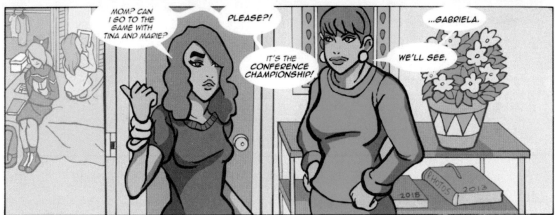

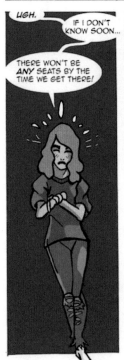

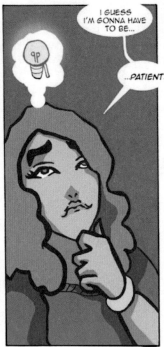

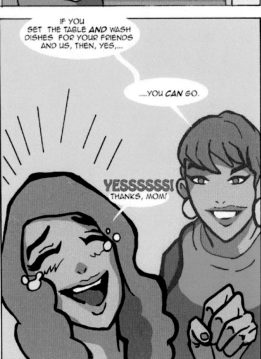

REFLECT

Gabriela and her mother had intuitive knowledge of what the statement "We'll see" meant. It meant that mom had the power in this situation. We don't know why she didn't want to give an answer right away—it might be she was distracted, or she wanted to tease Gabriella, or she needed to check on something or with someone else first. It really doesn't matter—it boiled down to Gabriella had to wait.

By spotting the real meaning, Gabriela knew why she was frustrated by her mother's answer—that she had to wait—and she could then react in a calm way instead of getting angry.

Gabriela's mother could have spotted that her reluctance to give an immediate answer would cause frustration to Gabriela, and she might have explained better when she would be able to give a more definite answer or what Gabriela might be able to do to get a yes answer. "I'll let you know after dinner," or "If you help me clean up after dinner, then you can go," are ways her mother could have immediately eased the frustration of not knowing.

If you are fully aware of something, then you can make plans to change it, to hold it back, or to express it—whichever is most appropriate and calming.

Spotting will help you choose whether to stay calm, make plans or take action. But it is difficult. Spotting requires thought, training, and practice until it becomes automatic.

ACTIVITY #1

Below write out a recent conflict with your parents or a friend where hidden meanings might have been at work. How did you react to what you thought was being said? How did you react to what was being expressed intuitively? What was your surface thinking and how did it influence your emotions and actions?

_____

_____

_____

_____

_____

_____

_____

Great! Now, let's take this same example and apply some tools to the situation above. What could you have done differently? How might it have influenced the outcome?

_____

_____

_____

_____

_____

_____

_____

Remember, spotting will help you stay calm, take action or make plans when you use it in the moment, but it takes work. It is difficult. You need to train with this technique and practice until it becomes second nature.

Here is how Gabriella used the 4-Step Method in this situation:

Step 1: I wanted to go to the game with my friends, and asked mom if it was OK. She said "We'll see," and that is when I started to get worked up.

Step 2: I was upset, I pouted, I worried I might not get to go, I wanted to cry or yell.

Step 3: I was angry that she didn't say OK right away, I was afraid she might not let me go. I spotted that I needed to be patient, that I didn't know what was on her mind, that I couldn't control her but I could control my reaction.

Step 4: Before using my tools, I would have cried or yelled at her that she was not being fair. We would have fought and she would have grounded me. Instead, I waited and she let me know that if I helped with supper then she would let me go to the game. I endorsed for staying calm.

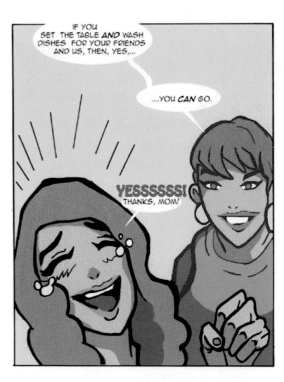

Humor

If you have an outburst of temper, and if you can see right away that the explosion is silly and laugh it off, then you are much less likely to have another outburst the next time you feel angry. Laughing it off relaxes you and gives you a way to defuse annoying incidents.

Humor isn't just about laughing—it can be an inner smile or a shrug. When you feel angry temper, try to shrug it off or find humor in the situation. When you are feeling fearful or insecure, use good humor to shake your head and change your reaction.

Earlier, Juan remembers that he used to live in constant temper. But now he has dropped his feeling of self-importance and developed a sense of humor. When he feels a friend is being rude by ignoring him, he makes an inner joke and laughs it off instead of blowing up.

Here is how Juan described his situation using the 4-Step Method:

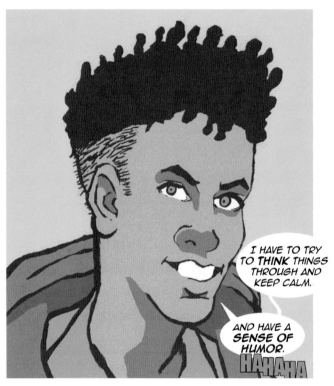

Step 1
I saw a friend at the coffee shop, and said hi, but he didn't hear me, so I called out again, and he yelled at me to leave him alone.

Step 2
I got hot, I scowled, I clenched my fists.

Step 3
I thought he was dissing me on purpose. Then I spotted that it was sort of silly—it didn't really matter, and he was just oblivious. I was proud I didn't lose my cool.

Step 4
Before using my tools, I would have yelled at him and told him off, and that would have been the end of our friendship. Now, I just shrugged and laughed it off.

Notice that he didn't report in his example the outcome that his friend apologized to him. He could have mentioned it, but the external outcome doesn't matter as much as his effort to control his temper. This is important to remember—regardless of how others react, it is how you use the tools and if they help you that matters.

ACTIVITY #2

Think of a time when you could have used humor to ease a tense situation. Describe it below:

_____

_____

_____

_____

What could have happened if you used humor?

_____

_____

_____

_____

We have spent a lot of time discussing how to manage an "angry" temper, but let's look at how we can manage a "fearful" one.

Face Your Fears

Remember, a fearful temper is often internally directed.

When things aren't going your way or a situation doesn't work out the way you planned you inflict damage on yourself. It could be physical, emotional, or in the form of self-talk. Whatever way it is expressed, the bottom line is that you often cannot tolerate discomfort and you take it out on yourself.

You blow off sports practice after a particularly bad game because you feel judged and self-critical. You are bored with your new job, so you ditch work. You aren't grasping history in your study group, so you blow off the exam.

All of these examples are fearful temper, where you "self-sabotage" rather than deal with the discomfort.

Face your Fears means going into the discomfort. It is not easy. It will be uncomfortable, challenging, scary, and awkward.

It is hard to go back to practice knowing that you bombed out the last game. It is difficult to put in the effort on a boring job when your friends are telling you to punch out and choose fun. It is challenging to make yourself study a subject you are not particularly good at or interested in.

When you face your fear you are better for it. The payoff isn't just overcoming that particular fear, but building a skill set that stays with you through the challenges and problems to come. That is a valuable lesson to learn from your fear.

ACTIVITY #3

In this section, we want you to think of a situation where you knew you were going to feel uncomfortable.

Maybe, you had to have a difficult conversation with a friend. Maybe, you had to own up to a mistake you made. Maybe, you had to go out of your comfort zone and speak in public, take on additional responsibility at your job, or tackle a project in school on a topic that you know nothing about.

In each of these situations, we are forced to choose between avoiding our fears or facing them head on.

Below, write a situation that happened in the past, where you were afraid you would make a mistake or fail, but you did it anyway. Write out how you successfully faced your fears and what the outcome looked like when you were done.

_____

_____

_____

_____

_____

_____

_____

_____

Okay, now look forward to the future. Choose an event, experience, challenge, or opportunity that you are afraid of tackling.

Use the 4-Step Method.

Write steps 1 and 2—describe the situation, describe your symptoms.

_____

_____

_____

_____

_____

_____

_____

_____

When you reach the spotting step of the 4-Step Method, make a choice to face your fear, use some of your tools, and see how the situation works out. Don't forget to endorse for the effort, regardless of outcome!

_____

_____

_____

_____

_____

_____

_____

_____

In the last chapter, we will talk about being group-minded instead of self-focused.

REVIEW

Wow. This is a lot to think about.

As with almost any skill, you get better at using it with practice. Don't look at this as just the end of the chapter, but as the beginning of putting these tools to work for you in life. As we conclude this section, you should know how to:

1. Look closer for Hidden Meanings behind statements and actions.

2. Use Humor as Tool to defuse anger.

3. Face your fears head on.

NOTES & THOUGHTS

GROUP MINDED VS. SELF-FOCUSED

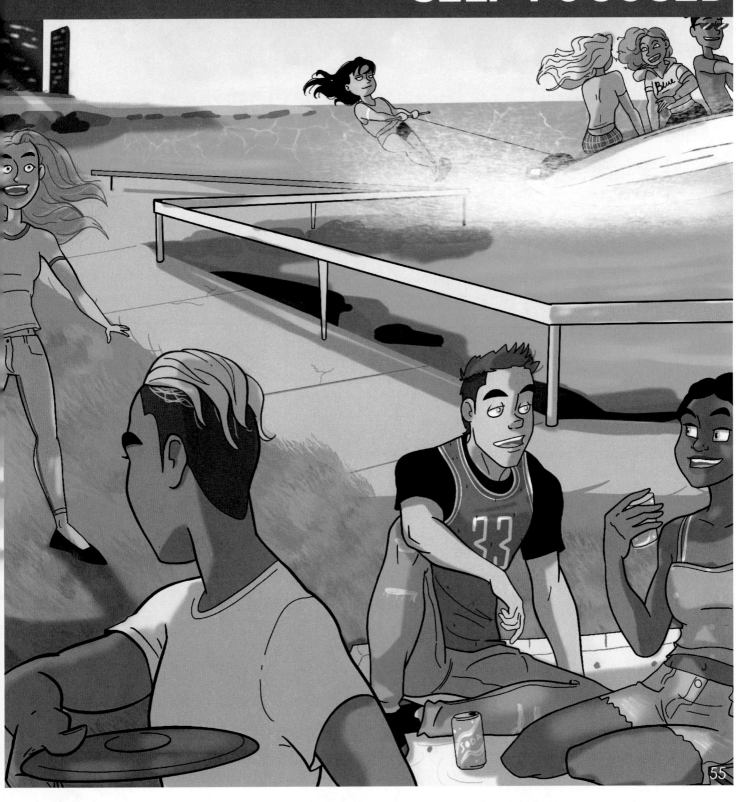

Part 7
GROUP MINDED VS. SELF-FOCUSED

IN THIS SECTION YOU WILL DISCOVER

1. We are all part of many groups
2. Importance of being group-minded over Self-Focused
3. Tools for Group-Mindedness

Congratulations!

You've reached the last chapter—what a journey it's been!

Group-Mindedness is the last concept we want to talk about.

It means service, self-control, and respect for the rights of others outside of yourself. What is also called fellowship.

We have spent a lot of time in previous chapters talking about how we cannot control others.

We have discussed how trying often leads to frustration. When we feel out of control ourselves and cannot manage our own emotions, we sometimes look to control those around us, which doesn't work very well!

The flipside of this is group-mindedness.

That is, respecting the autonomy and interests of the group, separate from ourselves and our own wants or needs.

Groups may be loosely connected—like a crowd at a concert—or close-knit, like a family.

All kinds of groups exist between the crowd and the family, with different degrees of fellowship. A group of friends should have far more fellowship than a group of students in a class at school, and the group of students in a class at school should have more fellowship than a group of strangers at a town meeting.

We are all part of many groups:

A family group.

A group of friends.

A class of students.

A sports team, band, choir or club.

Some have written rules, others don't.

But we must learn how to behave within each group or we will be unhappy and the group will not function well.

MEET ROBERT

He's got a lot on his mind, but when his mother asks him to run an errand, he's group-minded enough that he agrees, although grudgingly.

Then he runs into his girlfriend.

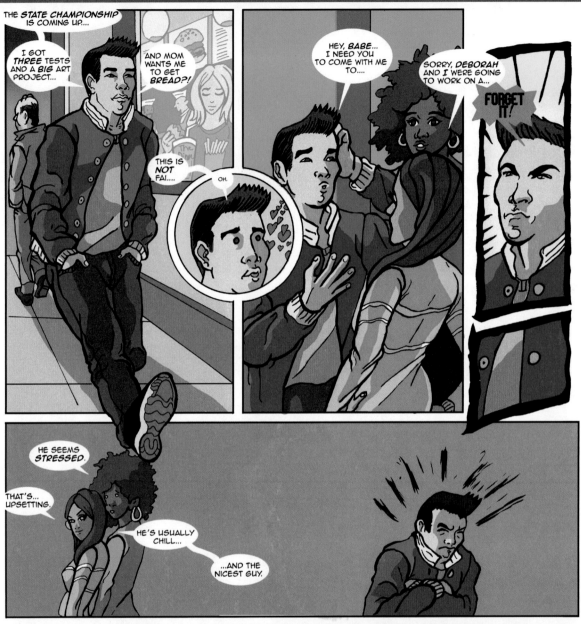

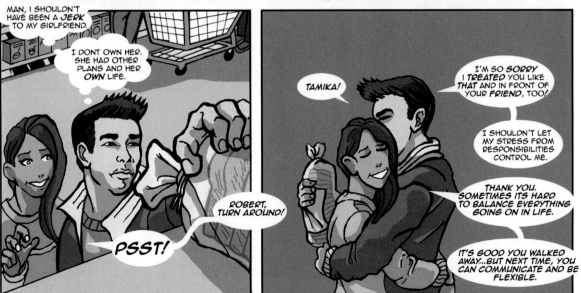

REFLECT

Before this program, Robert might have snapped at his mother for asking him to run an errand, but he agreed to do it for the sake of the family group.

People often forget the spirit of fellowship with their family and closest friends—temper is common in many families.

The same is true with boyfriends and girlfriends—one person might try to impose their will on the other. That's what Robert did at first, he demanded Tamika come with him—he didn't ask whether or not she had other plans, or invite her to join him.

But, by spotting that it is not necessary to dominate or compete, that it is helpful to be of service and group-minded at home and with friends, you will reduce temper and have more peace.

ACTIVITY #1

List all the groups that you are a part of below:
List your family, your school, your class, and your community.
List clubs, teams, organizations, and jobs.

_____   _____

_____   _____

_____   _____

_____   _____

Are there different expectations for how you act in each group?

To put it another way:

Do you act differently in school than when you are with your friends? How about when you are at a drama club meeting as opposed to a family dinner or picnic?

Write out how your own needs sometimes have to be put on hold for the needs of the group.

_____   _____

_____   _____

_____   _____

_____   _____

Here is Robert using the 4-Step Method:

Step 1: I was going to the store to get some bread for my mom, and I ran into my girlfriend and her friend. I wanted her to come with me, but she didn't want to...that's when I started getting worked up.

Step 2: I said "Forget it!" and stalked off. I was angry. I was clenching my jaw and fists.

Step 3: I spotted that I was being self-focused—I didn't even wait for her to really give me an answer. I was being demanding, not inviting her to come along. I totally ignored her friend, as if she didn't even exist—I was rude. I realized I was taking my frustration over having to run an errand out on my girlfriend. I started to calm down, and was thinking about what I should do.

Step 4: Before this program, I would have dwelled on my anger and felt that she had wronged me, not that I had done anything wrong. I would have kept up expecting her to drop everything when I showed up. Now I am more able to see her side, that she might have had plans with her friend, and that she didn't like me acting that way towards her. I endorsed for calming down and for not blaming her for my own actions.

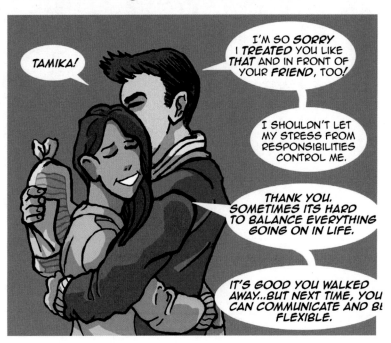

ACTIVITY #2

Review the tools below, and circle any others that you see in this example.

Some Tools for Group-Mindedness

- Don't take yourself too seriously.
- Be group-minded, not self-focused.
- People do things *that* annoy us, not *to* annoy us.
- Group-importance is favored over self-importance.
- Home should be the domain of service and cooperation.
- The feeling of fellowship gives rise to the will to peace.
- The will to peace makes for understanding, the will to power for misunderstanding.
- Don't cause offense and antagonize people.
- Seek balance in which group needs predominate over individualistic reactions without eliminating them.
- Common frustrations of daily life can be borne with a sense of humor.

This week, pay special attention to all the different groups in which you belong. Do you treat your family differently than your friends? Do you treat people you know differently than those you just met? Think about ways to maintain peace within each group, and how to be independent in constructive ways. Endorse for each effort to find balance in your groups and in your life.

REVIEW

As we conclude this section, you should know how to:

1. Apply Group-Mindedness in various situations.

2. Avoid being Self-Focused.

3. Have respect for the rights of others.

In the conclusion, we are going to look over everything that we've discussed and share some suggestions for continuing to build resilience.

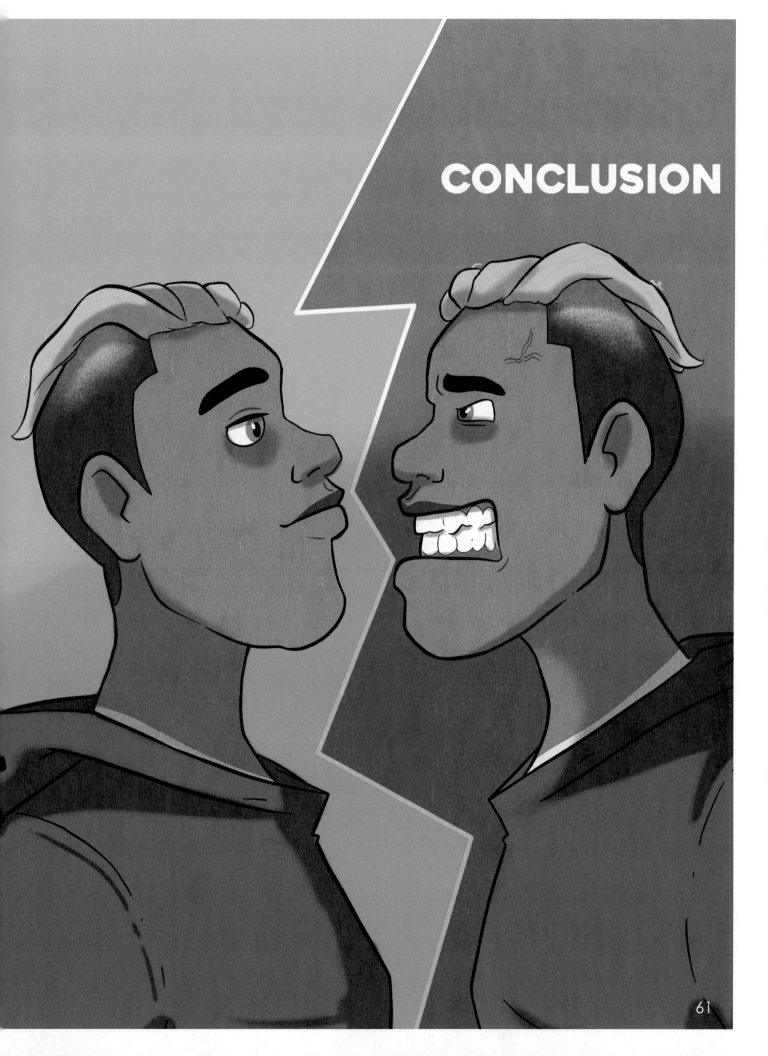

CONCLUSION

CONCLUSION

Congratulations!

You made it through the **Power Your Mind** program!

Hopefully this journey has been helpful, interesting, and informative. Most importantly, we hope you picked up some useful tools and skills along the way. Tools to help you with challenges and trivialities. Tools to help you manage your emotions, control your impulses, and handle events as they arise. Tools to **stop** negative thoughts and reactions, **think** about what is going on, and **do** something different that will make things better.

Remember: the number one expert on everything you are going through — is **you**!

In these pages you've learned:

- How your temper has two faces & what you can do about each.
- How you can handle situations outside of yourself and manage your internal thoughts and emotions.
- A Four-Step Method for handling trivial events.
- Lots of tools to deal with situations as they arise.
- And, much more!

Yes, it is a lot to think about and manage—that's why we wrote this book. It takes work to retrain your brain to think differently. What we are doing is called a cognitive-behavioral method—we help you use new words and concepts to teach your brain to become more resilient, to help you control your emotions and live a more peaceful and productive life.

Habits you develop today may help you not just tomorrow, but years down the road. The tools might pop into your head when you least expect them, and help you manage a tricky situation! Keep it up. Endorse.

Let's go back to page 2 where you started the session by looking over some of the success stories from other participants and developing your own personal goal. Take a moment to find that. Circle the rating that best describes how much progress you feel you have made toward that goal.

1	2	3	4	5	6	7	8	9	10
None at all									Much progress

Endorse yourself for the effort you've put toward that goal!

Keep this book on hand and with you in the weeks and months to come. Even though we have completed the program there is always more to learn. Revisit the exercises. Go back through the past sections to keep improving yourself. Learn new tools. Rework the activities. Try them out. Apply new tools to your life each time you work through this material.

In the next pages, you'll find a glossary of terms, resources, other books to help you on your journey, sample worksheets, and more. For more information on resources or to find Tools and 4-Step Method templates, go to **www.poweryourmind.org**.

Thank you! And, again, congrats.

GLOSSARY OF TERMS

We use specific words that have specific meanings—sometimes a little different than how these words would be in common usage. Using these words signals to your brain that you are thinking differently and that you are changing your thought patterns by using tools to stay calm.

Averageness: Most of daily life consists of average experiences that everyone faces. It is helpful to set realistic goals, and not expect perfection.

Group-minded: Thinking about what is best for your group (family, classmates, friends, etc.).

Bad Habits: Destructive behaviors that we do habitually and carelessly (i.e. crying habit, complaining habit, gossiping habit, sarcasm habit).

Good Habits: Endorsing, using our tools, exercising, being group-minded, etc.

Inner Environment: Everything inside oneself including feelings, sensations, thoughts, and impulses.

Feelings: Emotions such as anger, impatience, hatred, fear, worry, embarrassment, shame, and many more. You cannot control your initial feelings.

Sensations: Physical responses such as blushing, racing heartbeats, tense muscles, teary eyes, and many more. You cannot control these initial sensations.

Thoughts: Ideas produced by thinking, such as, "This is fun," "I can do this," "He is annoying," and so on. You can learn to change your thoughts.

Impulses: What you first want to do, such as to punch, to run, to hug, to laugh, to yell, and so on. You can learn to control your impulses.

Outer Environment: Everything outside oneself, including people, the weather, traffic, events, and the past.

Sabotage: Anything done to interfere with the goal of managing anger and fear, such as using temperamental language, not using the tools, or rebelling. When we ignore or choose not to practice what we have learned. When we do not do what is best for our mental health.

Self-endorsement: A mental "pat on the back," self-praise for effort in practicing the method, using tools, and controlling thoughts and impulses; recognizing the value of every effort regardless of the result.

Self-Focused: Asserting individual rights and domination over someone else.

Spotting: Identifying a disturbing feeling, sensation, thought or impulse; then applying the tools. Understanding the underlying meaning of words or events, and using tools to react.

Symptoms: Thoughts or physical reactions to fearful or angry temper (i.e. lethargy, agitation, increased heart rate).

Temper: Caused by judging right and wrong in minor, everyday events. (Note: This does not apply to legal, moral, or ethical issues.)

Angry Temper: Negative judgments directed against another person or situation (i.e. they are wrong). This can take the form of resentment, impatience, indignation, annoyance, irritation, disgust, hatred or rebellion.

Fearful Temper: Negative judgments directed against oneself (i.e. I am wrong). This can take the form of discouragement, preoccupation, worry, embarrassment, hopelessness or despair.

Temperamental deadlock: Quarreling over who is right and who is wrong in everyday situations—it doesn't matter! It becomes an angry standoff.

Temperamental language: Exaggerated, negative, or insecure descriptions of experiences. All language that is alarming and defeating.

Tools: Short sentences or phrases that are used as reminders of the techniques and concepts we are learning and practicing.

Trivialities: The routine events and irritations of daily life. Most events are trivial when compared to the importance of our health (mental, spiritual, emotional and physical).

Vicious cycle: Temper and tenseness that increase the length and intensity of negative feelings and sensations.

Vitalizing Cycle: Developing positive emotions and thoughts, leading to a greater sense of vitality, peace, security and confidence.

Will: The power to choose how you are going to act and what you are going to think.

Working ourselves up: When we take negative or distressing thoughts and impulses and escalate them.

Working ourselves down: Using tools to change reactions, relieve tension, reduce anxiety or temper, or become calm.

RESOURCES

In addition to this workbook and other publications, **Recovery International** offers many ways to participate in support groups to practice giving examples and using your tools.

Community Meetings: Weekly meetings are held in communities throughout the country run by trained peer leaders who will assist you in learning how to spot and give examples. Affiliates in Canada, Ireland and Puerto Rico also offer meetings.

Telephone Meetings: Weekly telephone meetings are available for members who cannot attend community meetings, or who wish to supplement other meetings. Newcomer training is required to practice the method and learn telephone meeting protocol, and then you will be able to participate in an assigned meeting.

Online Meetings: Online meetings offer the benefit of attending from your own home, and allow for interaction with the leader and other participants through screen sharing readings and spots.

Chat Meetings: Chat meetings enable you to post examples and spot on others' examples through moderated yet informal chat format postings.

Facebook Meetings Page: This closed group page allows you to post examples and spot on others' examples 24/7 in a moderated setting.

You can find more information about membership and meeting schedules on our website at **www.recoveryinternational.org**. We invite you to seek out a group meeting near you, or consider Leader Training to open a meeting in your community!

This workbook is designed to be used as a self-help program or part of a group training session. While the Recovery International Method often serves as an adjunct to professional care, it is not a substitute for therapy, counseling or medical advice. If you believe you need such counseling or advice, please contact a mental health or health care professional.

Final thought:

This method works for many people, but it takes a lot of time, effort and practice. You have to retrain your brain to use the tools and react differently to everyday situations. Often, it takes five or six weekly meetings to learn the method and even longer to know the tools well enough to apply them in everyday situations. So, give yourself enough time to try it out, practice spotting and the four-step method, and let it work for you.

Books by and about Dr. Abraham Low and Recovery International

The origins and ideas behind the tools and this method can be found in the following books:

Mental Health Through Will Training by Abraham Low, M.D.– Primary text of Low's work used at Recovery International meetings. (First published 1950; Fourth Edition, 2019.)

Selections from Dr. Low's Work by Abraham Low, M.D. – Writings from 1950 to 1953 that include additional insights for practicing the Recovery International Method. (Published in full,1953; Third Edition, 2019.)

Manage Your Fears, Manage Your Anger by Abraham Low, M.D.– Transcriptions of Low's 70 taped lectures from 1953 and 1954. (First published 1995; Third Edition, 2019.)

Peace vs. Power In The Family: Domestic Discord and Emotional Distress by Abraham Low, M.D.– Writings focused on family dynamics. (First published as Lectures to Relatives of Former Patients, 1943; Third Edition, 2014.)

Mental Illness, Stigma and Self-Help, The Founding of Recovery, Inc. – Describes the early development of Recovery International. (First published as The Historical Development of Recovery's Self-Help Project, 1943; Second Edition, 1991)

My Dear Ones, Neil and Margaret Rau – Biography of Dr. Abraham Low and Recovery International. (First published 1971; Reprinted 1990)

The Wisdom of Dr. Low – Compilation of Low's inspiring words in an easy reference format to help with a current problem or for daily affirmations. (First Published 2009; Second Edition 2019.)

RI Discovery Workbook – Workbook used at RI Discovery meetings, including selected re-written chapters of Low's works. (First Published 2009; Third Edition 2019)

For more information or to support the Better. Mental. Health.™ programs of Recovery International visit www.recoveryinternational.org.

EXAMPLE WORKSHEET

Step 1: Report a situation—an everyday event when you began to work yourself up. Describe what happened: specifically, what triggered temper and symptoms?

_____

_____

_____

Step 2: Report the symptoms you experienced—both physical and mental. (For instance, angry and fearful thoughts, confusion, tightness in your chest, low feelings, sweaty palms, and so on.)

_____

_____

_____

How would you rate your discomfort on a scale of 1 to 10? (1 mild to 10 very intense)

Before Spotting: 1   2   3   4   5   6   7   8   9   10

Step 3: Report your spotting of fearful and/or angry temper, the RI tools you used to help yourself, and self-endorsement for your effort.

_____

_____

_____

Step 4: Describe what would have happened before your training—the reaction and discomfort you would have experienced:

_____

_____

_____

Rate your reaction and symptoms after using the tools in this program on a scale of 1 to 10.

After Spotting: 1   2   3   4   5   6   7   8   9   10

Endorse yourself for your effort or any improvement!

EXAMPLE WORKSHEET

Step 1: Report a situation—an everyday event when you began to work yourself up. Describe what happened: specifically, what triggered temper and symptoms?

_____

_____

_____

Step 2: Report the symptoms you experienced—both physical and mental. (For instance, angry and fearful thoughts, confusion, tightness in your chest, low feelings, sweaty palms, and so on.)

_____

_____

_____

How would you rate your discomfort on a scale of 1 to 10? (1 mild to 10 very intense)

Before Spotting: 1 2 3 4 5 6 7 8 9 10

Step 3: Report your spotting of fearful and/or angry temper, the RI tools you used to help yourself, and self-endorsement for your effort.

_____

_____

_____

Step 4: Describe what would have happened before your training—the reaction and discomfort you would have experienced:

_____

_____

_____

_____

Rate your reaction and symptoms after using the tools in this program on a scale of 1 to 10.

After Spotting: 1 2 3 4 5 6 7 8 9 10

Endorse yourself for your effort or any improvement!

EXAMPLE WORKSHEET

Step 1: Report a situation—an everyday event when you began to work yourself up. Describe what happened: specifically, what triggered temper and symptoms?

_____

_____

_____

Step 2: Report the symptoms you experienced—both physical and mental. (For instance, angry and fearful thoughts, confusion, tightness in your chest, low feelings, sweaty palms, and so on.)

_____

_____

_____

How would you rate your discomfort on a scale of 1 to 10? (1 mild to 10 very intense)

Before Spotting: 1 2 3 4 5 6 7 8 9 10

Step 3: Report your spotting of fearful and/or angry temper, the RI tools you used to help yourself, and self-endorsement for your effort.

_____

_____

_____

Step 4: Describe what would have happened before your training—the reaction and discomfort you would have experienced:

_____

_____

_____

_____

Rate your reaction and symptoms after using the tools in this program on a scale of 1 to 10.

After Spotting: 1 2 3 4 5 6 7 8 9 10

Endorse yourself for your effort or any improvement!

EXAMPLE WORKSHEET

Step 1: Report a situation—an everyday event when you began to work yourself up. Describe what happened: specifically, what triggered temper and symptoms?

_____

_____

_____

Step 2: Report the symptoms you experienced—both physical and mental. (For instance, angry and fearful thoughts, confusion, tightness in your chest, low feelings, sweaty palms, and so on.)

_____

_____

_____

How would you rate your discomfort on a scale of 1 to 10? (1 mild to 10 very intense)

Before Spotting: 1   2   3   4   5   6   7   8   9   10

Step 3: Report your spotting of fearful and/or angry temper, the RI tools you used to help yourself, and self-endorsement for your effort.

_____

_____

_____

Step 4: Describe what would have happened before your training—the reaction and discomfort you would have experienced:

_____

_____

_____

Rate your reaction and symptoms after using the tools in this program on a scale of 1 to 10.

After Spotting: 1   2   3   4   5   6   7   8   9   10

Endorse yourself for your effort or any improvement!

Made in the USA
Coppell, TX
23 December 2022

90580937R00045